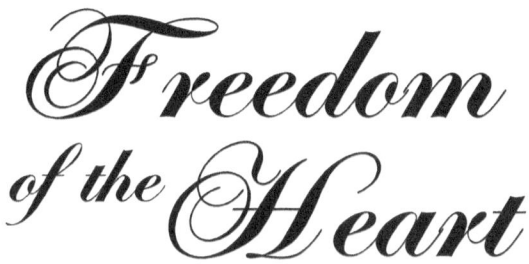

Freedom of the Heart

A JOURNEY BACK TO INNOCENCE
THROUGH THE
EYES OF A YOUNG ADULT WITH
DOWN SYNDROME

Ana Agostini
for
Gabriel Hernandez

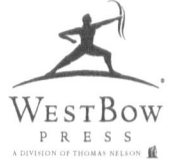

WESTBOW
PRESS
A DIVISION OF THOMAS NELSON

WestBow Press books may be ordered through booksellers or by contacting:

WestBow Press
A Division of Thomas Nelson
1663 Liberty Drive
Bloomington, IN 47403
www.westbowpress.com
1-(866) 928-1240

Because of the dynamic nature of the Internet, any web addresses or links contained in this book may have changed since publication and may no longer be valid. The views expressed in this work are solely those of the author and do not necessarily reflect the views of the publisher, and the publisher hereby disclaims any responsibility for them.

Any people depicted in stock imagery provided by Thinkstock are models, and such images are being used for illustrative purposes only.

Certain stock imagery © Thinkstock.

ISBN: 978-1-4497-7107-2 (sc)
ISBN: 978-1-4497-7108-9 (e)

Library of Congress Control Number: 2012919228

Printed in the United States of America

WestBow Press rev. date: 10/17/2012

GABY CALLED HIS DRAWING
FREEDOM OF THE HEART AND
IT LATER BECAME THE TITLE
OF THIS BOOK.

Biography

Ana Agostini is a teacher of Students with Special Needs committed with God, her family, and community service. Ana is the dedicated mother of Gabriel, and Anais.

After dealing with a severe depression of her oldest son, she turned a challenging situation into hope for others by publishing this devotional guide of emotional freedom.

She believes that everything happens for a reason, and the reason is to proclaim victory through God's UNCONDITIONAL love.

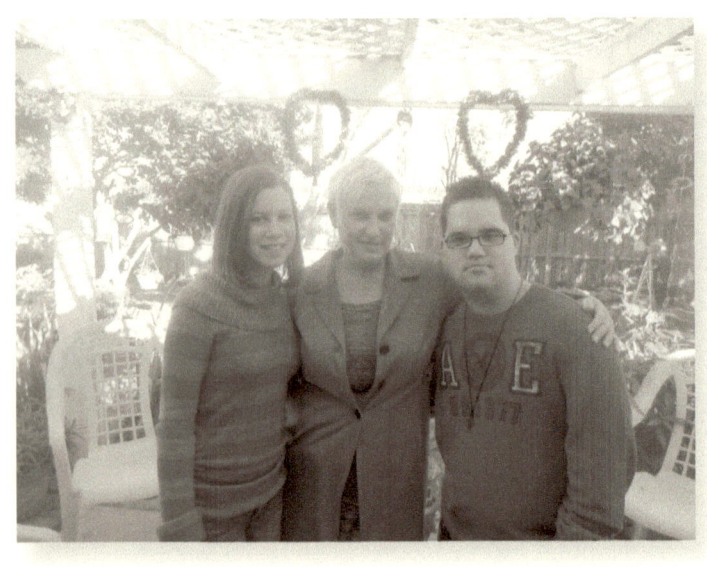

From left to right, Anais, Ana and Gaby.

Special Thanks

First of all, this book is dedicated to God. He is the one that gives us the strength, faith and wisdom to never give up during the journey. His inspiration to leave a legacy to others is priceless.

Second, I would like to dedicate this book to all the parents of kids with disabilities for their unconditional love to them, their warrior hearts and resilience.

Third, I would like to express my gratitude to the collaboration of the artists Wilson Romero, Julio Sanchez, and Alexis Artuna for being able to transfer Gaby's words to a canvas.

This book has been made possible by the financial contribution of Ibrahim and Melba Silwany in alliance with Gloria Puerto from Feed and Fortify Community Organization.

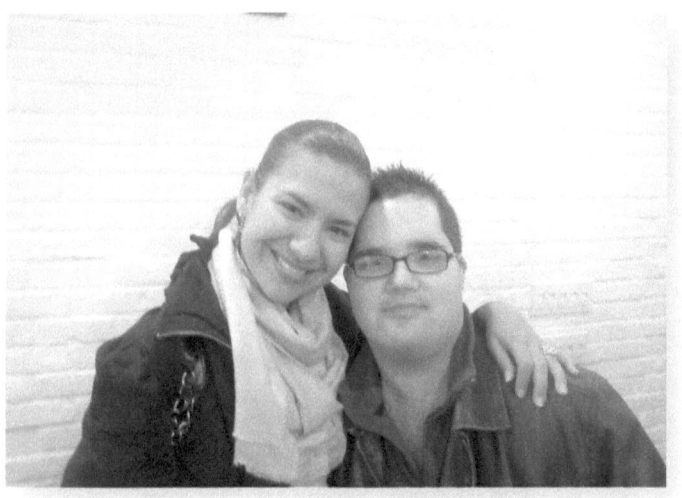

THANKS TO GLORIA PUERTO FROM FEED AND FORTIFY COMMUNITY ORGANIZATION FOR BELIEVING IN THIS VISION.

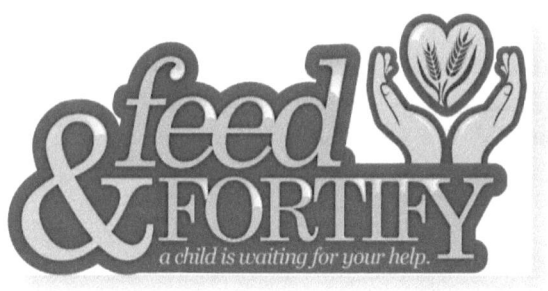

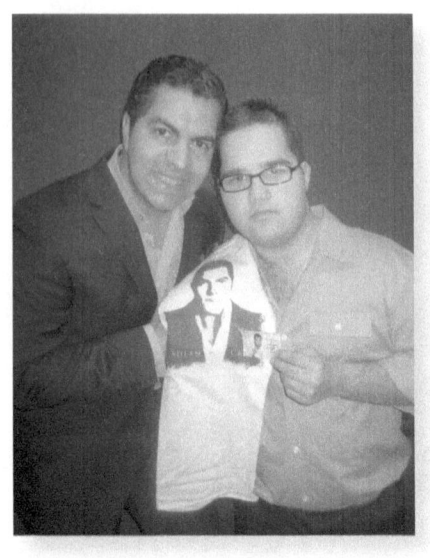

Also, thanks to the Christian Puerto Rican pianist, composer and producer Adlan Cruz and his Foundation for sharing his vision of this devotional for the glory of God.

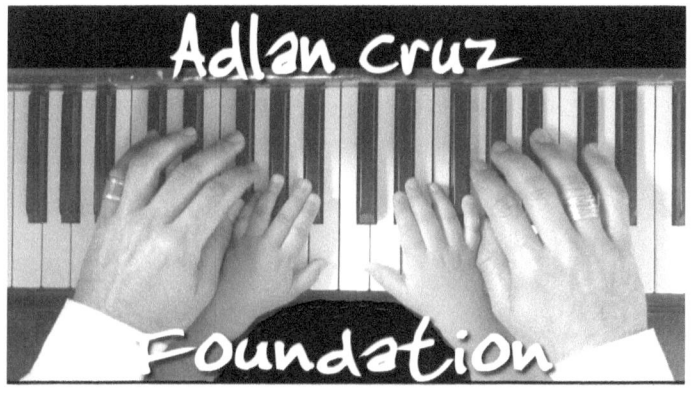

For more information go to

adlancruzfoundation.com

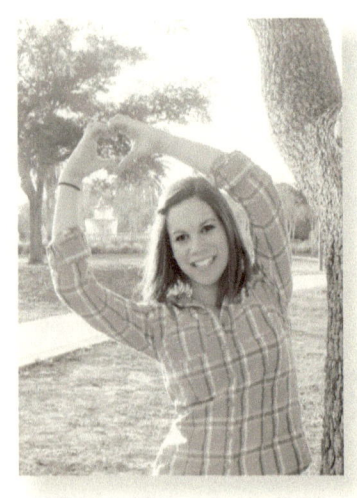

ANAIS LOVES HER BROTHER VERY MUCH. DURING THE CRISIS OF HIS DEPRESSION SHE ASKED GOD TO RETURN HER BROTHER BACK TO HER. SHE IS GREATFUL HE DID.

SHE WAS ALSO INSPIRED TO WRITE THIS ESSAY SHE TITLED;

FROM A SISTER'S HEART

FROM A SISTER'S HEART BY ANAIS HERNANDEZ

An African proverb says; "It takes two parents to produce a child, but it takes a whole village to raise the child." A significant person in my life is my big brother. My brother has helped me to become more mature for my age, by helping me to see the world in a different (positive) way. This is due to his condition.

Another way that my brother has helped me to grow as a human being is the following; He always tells me when I just out of nowhere start crying, he tells me "I'm here for you" or "Be happy".

To add on to that, I see my brother like a positive light. I sometimes think my brother has interpersonal intelligence. My reason for that is because every time he notices that someone is sad, he tells that person many positive messages.

I barely see my brother sad or angry. If I do, it is very rare that he would be. When I look at my brother and I am feeling sad or angry, I think, if my brother that has Down syndrome is very tough, then why can't I be like him?

My big brother gives me strength and faith.

In conclusion, I love my brother very much. He is a person that I think everyone should look up to. I personally think that my brother was brought to life by God on October 26, 1988, to bring a message of Love, Faith, and Peace to this world.

How to read this book

Each chapter is dedicated to a different topic. On each page, you will find Gaby's affirmation quoted first, then, the bible scripture related to the affirmation and my personal reflection of Gaby's transformation at the bottom. Enjoy!

Table of Contents

Chapter 1: God 1

Chapter 2: Heart 19

Chapter 3: Jesus 33

Chapter 4: Love 63

Chapter 5: Angels 69

Chapter 6: Freedom 77

Chapter 7: Random Wisdom
            from A Pure Heart.. 83

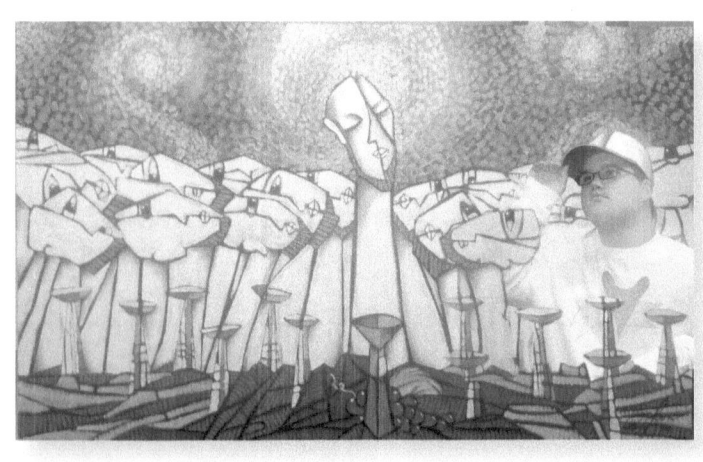

Art by Wilson Romero

GOD

CHAPTER ONE

John 4:24

Gaby's journey has brought

him into a close encounter

with God. Here is how he

describes Him.

1. Gaby: "The power of God is love"

1 John 4:16
And so we know and rely on the love God has for us. God is love. Whoever lives in love lives in God, and God in him.

Mom: Love is the power that moves humans to take action and is inspiration that comes from God. He has given me a tool to become my son's coach in his challenging journey of self-discovery.

2. Gaby: "God is kingdom"

Luke 17:21

Nor will people say, 'Here it is, or there it is,' because the kingdom of God is within you."

Mom: Gaby has discovered the kingdom of God connection inside him through the freedom of his heart, his inner peace and his faith.

3. Gaby: "God takes care of me"

Psalm 31:7
I will be glad and rejoice in your love, for you saw my affliction and knew the anguish of my soul.

Mom: Gaby takes refuge in God.

4. Gaby: "God is open"

James 1:5

If any of you lacks wisdom, he should ask God, who gives generously to all without finding fault, and it will be given to him.

Mom: Gaby expresses God's availability to all.

5. Gaby: "Energy of God is love"

John 4:24

For God is Spirit, so those who worship him must worship in spirit and in truth.

Mom: Gaby identifies God's love as a powerful energy that you cannot see but feel.

6. Gaby: "God is the Sun"

Revelation 22:16

"I, Jesus, have sent my angel to give you this testimony for the churches. I am the Root and the offspring of David, and the bright Morning Star."

Mom: Gaby identifies God with the light of the sun.

7. Gaby: "The power of God is in this home"

Genesis 28: 17
How awesome is this place! This is none other than the house of God; this is the gate of heaven.

Mom: Gaby can feel God's presence in his home. We all can feel that when we engage in worship and prayer.

8. Gaby: "God is the king"

Psalm 47:7

For *God is the King* of all the earth; sing to him a psalm of praise.

Mom: Gaby identifies God's authority.

9. Gaby: "God wins"

Psalm 60:12

With *God* we will gain the victory, and he will trample down our enemies.

Mom: Gaby knows there is a spiritual warfare going on. He also knows who wins.

10. Gaby: "God loves me, alleluia!"

Philippians 3:1
The joy of the Lord is my strength. In the days of trial and tribulation seek my joy for I am you Savior and will deliver you from these tough times praising God even when things aren't going good.

Mom: Gaby exalts God's love. He can reach His throne.

11. Gaby: "God is watching you here" (pointing to his heart)

Jeremiah 29: 11-13
For I know the plans I have for you," declares the Lord, "plans to prosper you and not to harm you, plans to give you hope and a future. Then you will call on me and come and pray to me, and I will listen to you. You will seek me and find me when you seek me with all your heart.

Mom: Gaby's relationship and connection with God reveals the door, the heart.

12. Gaby: "God is happy, glory!"

Psalm 63:5
I will be fully satisfied as with the richest of foods; with singing lips my mouth will praise you.

Mom: Gaby is praising.

13. Gaby: "Kingdom of God, freedom of the heart"

1 Corinthians 3:16

Don't you know that you yourselves are God's temple and that God's Spirit dwells in your midst?

Mom: Gaby's connection with God's kingdom is through his inner peace and his faith in Him.

14. Gaby: "Holy, holy"

Isaiah 6:3

They were calling out to each other, "Holy, holy, holy is the LORD of Heaven's Armies! The whole earth is filled with his glory!"

Mom: Gaby enters into His presence by praising again.

15. Gaby: "God is good"

1 Chronicles 16:34

Give thanks to the lord, for he is good; his love endures forever.

Mom: God is good, all the time.

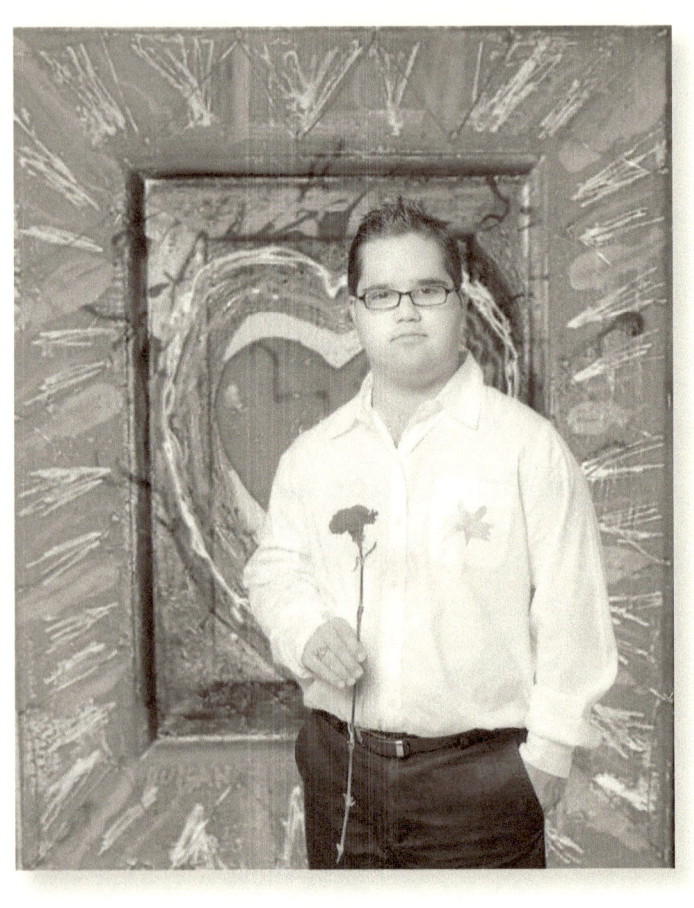

Art by Julio Sanchez-JULSAN

HEART

CHAPTER TWO

1Timothy 1:5

My son's heart was broken
to a point where he was
expressing that it was closed
and bleeding. In this chapter,
Gaby expresses freedom from
his captive soul in his own
perception.

1. Gaby: "My heart is normal"

Psalm 51:10

Create in me a pure *heart*, O God, and renew a steadfast spirit within me.

Mom: Inner peace makes his heart normal. He is able to know the difference between sadness and relief.

2. Gaby: "Be free, open your heart and relax"

Phillipians 4:8-9

Finally, brothers and sisters, whatever is true, whatever is noble, whatever is right, whatever is pure, whatever is lovely, whatever is admirable if anything is excellent or praiseworthy think about such things. Whatever you have learned or received or heard from me, or seen in me put it into practice. And the God of peace will be with you.

Mom: In order to receive God's peace, we must be willing to receive it by releasing the blocks and by changing our thoughts into a positive mind set.

3. Gaby: "Everybody loves me in my heart"

1 Peter 3:8

Finally, all of you, be like-minded, be sympathetic, *love one another*, and be compassionate and humble.

Mom: Gaby can feel the empathy of others toward him during his process. Support from love ones is key for recovery.

4. Gaby: "Freedom of the heart, white heart"

Matthew 5:8
Blessed are the pure in heart, for they will see God.

Mom: Gaby identifies his freedom through a pure heart. White symbolizes purity.

5. Gaby: "My heart is peace"

1Timothy 1:5

The purpose of my instruction is that all believers would be filled with love that comes from a pure heart, a clear conscience, and genuine faith.

Mom: Freedom in his heart translates to peace. As Gaby's self-confidence gets a boost, he feels empowered.

6. Gaby: "I am free, in my heart"

Psalms 51:10
Create in me a clean heart, O God, and renew a right spirit within me.

Mom: Gaby no longer feels captive.

7. Gaby: "My heart is the king"

Ephesians 3: 16-17

I pray that out of his glorious riches he may strengthen you with power through his Spirit in your inner being, so that Christ may dwell in your hearts through faith.

Mom: After recognizing Jesus as the king, Gaby embraces His attributes of unconditional love by faith.

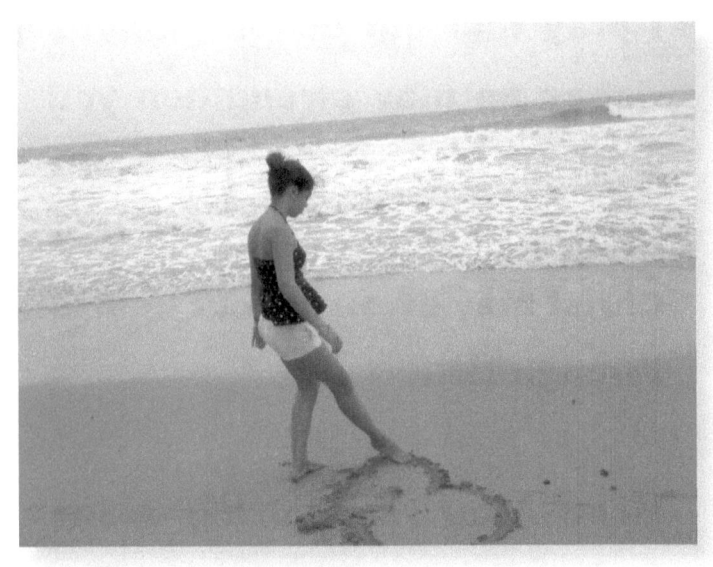

God is love

8. Gaby: "Follow your heart"

Ecclesiastes 11:9

You who are young, be happy while you are young, and let your *heart* give you joy in the days of your youth. *Follow* the ways of your *heart* and whatever your eyes see, but know that for all these things God will bring you into judgment.

Mom: Whatever our heart tells us to do, we do, but beware sometimes our heart can fool us. Make sure you follow God's guidance.

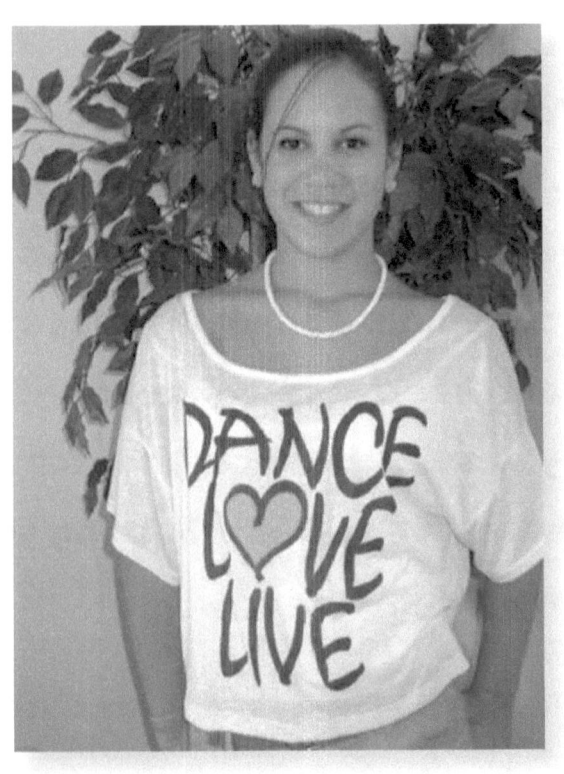

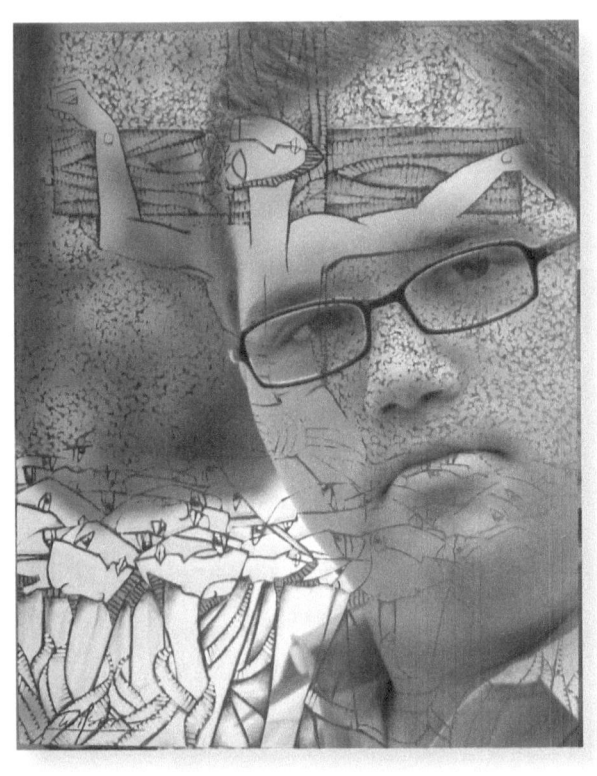

Art by Wilson Romero

JESUS

CHAPTER THREE

John 3:16

My son enters into an intimate relationship with Jesus to a point where it seems he is able to see him.

1. Gaby: "Jesus is light"

John 8:12

When *Jesus* spoke again to the people, he said, "I am the *light* of the world. Whoever follows me will never walk in darkness, but will have the *light* of life."

Mom: Once free, we can get out of the darkness through Jesus.

2. Gaby: "Power of love, the king"

Revelation 19:16

On his robe and on his thigh he has this name written: *king* of kings and lord of lords.

Mom: Gaby recognizes Jesus as the king.

3. Gaby: "Jesus is the Lord"

1 Corinthians 1:3

Grace and peace to you from God our Father and the *Lord Jesus* Christ.

Mom: Gaby recognizes Jesus as the lord of lords.

4. Gaby: "The king is open"

Matthew 7:7

Ask and it will be given to you; seek and you will find; *knock* and the door will be opened to you.

Mom: Gaby expresses Jesus' availability to all.

5. Gaby: "Jesus' father is God"

Hebrews 5:5

In the same way, Christ did not take on himself the glory of becoming a high priest. But God said to him, you are my Son; today I have become your Father.

Mom: Gaby recognizes Jesus as the son of God

6. Gaby: "Jesus is in heaven to pray me"

John 14:6
Jesus answered, "I am the way and the truth and the life. No one comes to the Father except through me.

Mom: Jesus is the way to the Father.

7. Gaby: "Believe in Jesus"

John 12:44

Then *Jesus* cried out, "Whoever believes in me does not believe in me only, but in the one who sent me.

Mom: Gaby is preaching.

8. Gaby: "Jesus, my cross"

Matthew 16:24

Then *Jesus* said to his disciples, "Whoever wants to be my disciple must deny themselves and take up their *cross* and follow me.

Mom: Gaby relates his affliction with Jesus' calvary.

9. Gaby: "My mama says: Jesus loves me"

2 Timothy 3:15
...and how from infancy you have known the Holy Scriptures, which are able to make you wise for salvation through faith in Christ *Jesus*.

Mom: As parents, we must introduce Jesus to our children.

10. Gaby: "Jesus is the power of God"

Galatians 4:6
Because you are his sons, God sent the Spirit of his Son into our hearts.

Mom: Gaby recognizes Jesus as the energy of love into our hearts.

11. Gaby: "My key is Jesus. Kingdom of God, freedom"

Matthew 22:2
The kingdom of heaven is like a king who prepared a wedding banquet for his son.

Mom: Faith in Jesus is the key that opens the gates to the kingdom of God.

12. Gaby: "Jesus, my cross in my heart"

1st John 4:4

You, dear children, are from God and have overcome them, because the one who is in you is greater than the one who is in the world.

Mom: Gaby knows Jesus lives in his heart like the cross he wears.

13. Gaby: "Jesus is out there"

1 John 2:1

My dear children, I write this to you so that you will not sin. But if anybody does sin, we have one who speaks to the Father in our defense Jesus Christ, the Righteous One.

Mom: Gaby understands the availability to reach for Jesus at any time.

14. Gaby: "Jesus is the king"

Revelation 19:16

On his robe and on his thigh he has this name written: *king of kings* and lord of lords.

Mom: Gaby recognizes the king of kings.

15. Gaby: "Power is Jesus"

John 13:3

Jesus knew that the Father had put all things under his *power*, and that he had come from God and was returning to God.

Mom: Gaby believes in a powerful God.

16. Gaby:" Jesus is a hero"

1 Corinthians 15:57

But thanks are to God! He gives us the victory through our Lord *Jesus* Christ.

Mom: Gaby recognizes Jesus as our deliverer.

17. Gaby: "My life is Jesus"

1 John 4:15

If anyone acknowledges that *Jesus* is the Son of God, God lives in them and them in God.

Mom: Gaby acknowledges Jesus' attributes in his life.

18. Gaby: "Jesus is around"

1 Corinthians 16:23

The grace of the Lord *Jesus* be with you.

Mom: Gaby feels His presence, His grace.

19. Gaby: "Love is Jesus' peace"

Ephesians 3:16-19
I pray that out of his glorious riches he may strengthen you with power through his Spirit in your inner being, so that Christ may dwell in your hearts through faith. And I pray that you, being rooted and established in love, may have power, together with all the Lord's holy people, to grasp how wide and long and high and deep is the love of Christ, and to know this love

that surpasses knowledge that you may be filled to the measure of all the fullness of God.

Mom: Gaby enters into God's rest through the love of Jesus.

20. Gaby: "Every day, Jesus comes first"

Romans 1:8

First, I thank my God through Jesus Christ for all of you, because your faith is being reported all over the world.

Mom: When we give priority to Jesus into our lives every day, we can experience inner peace.

21. Gaby: "Blood of Jesus"

Hebrews 10:19

Therefore, brothers and sisters, since we have confidence to enter the Most Holy Place by the *blood of Jesus*,

Mom: Gaby recognizes the power of Jesus' sacrifice.

22. Gaby: "Jesus, open the windows in heaven"

Hebrews 4:16
Let us then approach God's throne of grace with confidence, so that we may receive mercy and find grace to help us in our time off.

Mom: Jesus is the key that gives us access to God's throne.

23. Gaby: "Jesus is the flower"

Solomon 2:1

"I am the rose of Sharon, and the lily of the valleys."

Jesus is symbolically referred to as the rose of Sharon. Jesus is perfect in His God nature.

Bible: Article Source:
http://EzineArticles.com/20007

24. Gaby: "Jesus is in heaven, real love. Heaven is Jesus"

Luke 24:51
While he was blessing them, he left them and was taken up into *heaven*.

Mom: Gaby recognizes Jesus in the gates of heaven.

25. Gaby: "Jesus made me free"

Galatians 5:1

Stand fast therefore in the liberty with which Christ has made us free, and be not entangled again with the yoke of bondage.

Mom: Gaby finds freedom through Jesus.

26. Gaby: "The power of God is Jesus in your body and your soul"

Galatians 4:6
Because you are his sons, God sent the Spirit of his Son into our hearts, the Spirit who calls out, Abba Father. So you are no longer a slave, but God's child; and since you are his child, God has made you also an heir.

Mom: Gaby describes the Holy Spirit as Jesus' spirit inside us.

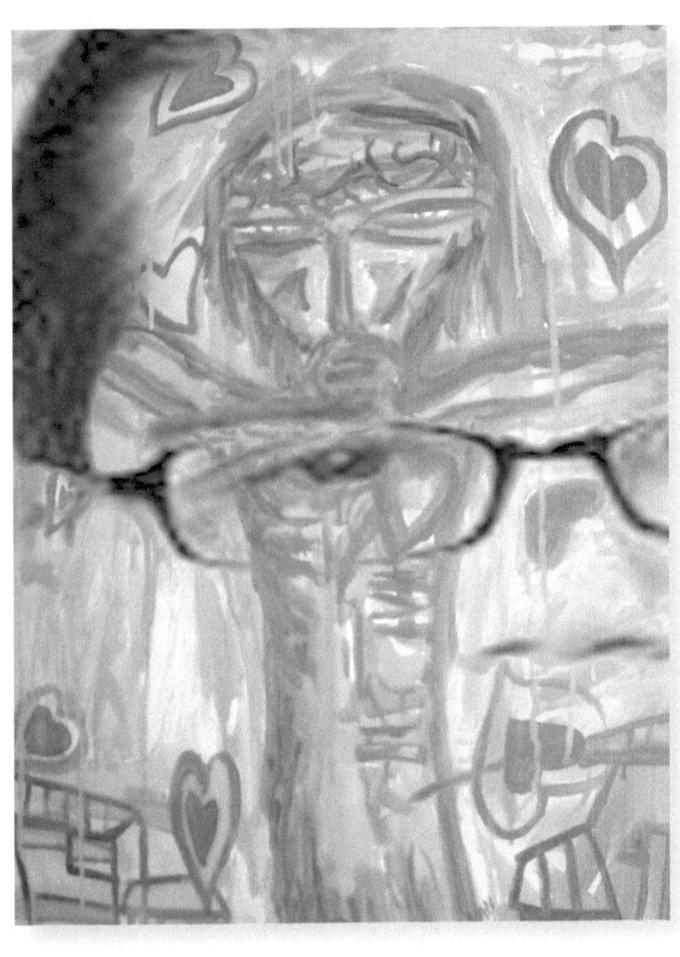

Art by Julio Sanchez-JULSAN

LOVE

CHAPTER FOUR

1 Corinthians 13:13
Love is the ultimate
expression of God for He is
love. Love endures all things
and Gaby gives it many
definitions.

Gaby says:

1. "Love is open"

2. "Love is power"

3. "Mother and son is AMORE"

4. "Love is AMORE"

5. "Love is happiness"

6. "Gloria is love"

7. "Power of love

8. "Love, happiness is angel wings"

9. "True love is Jesus"

10. "My mom loves me"

11. "My cousin loves me"

12. "My sister loves me"

13. "My mom loves me, my friends, and my best buddy"

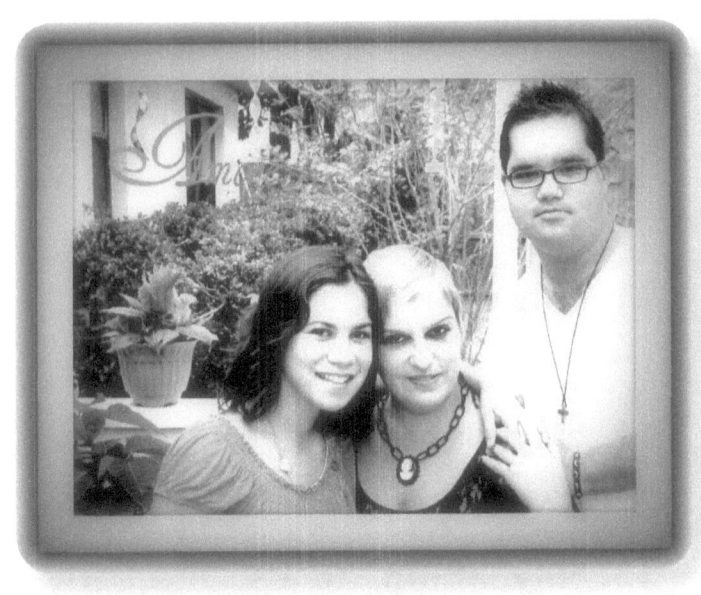

**FAITH, HOPE, LOVE, AND THE
GREATEST OF THESE IS LOVE.**

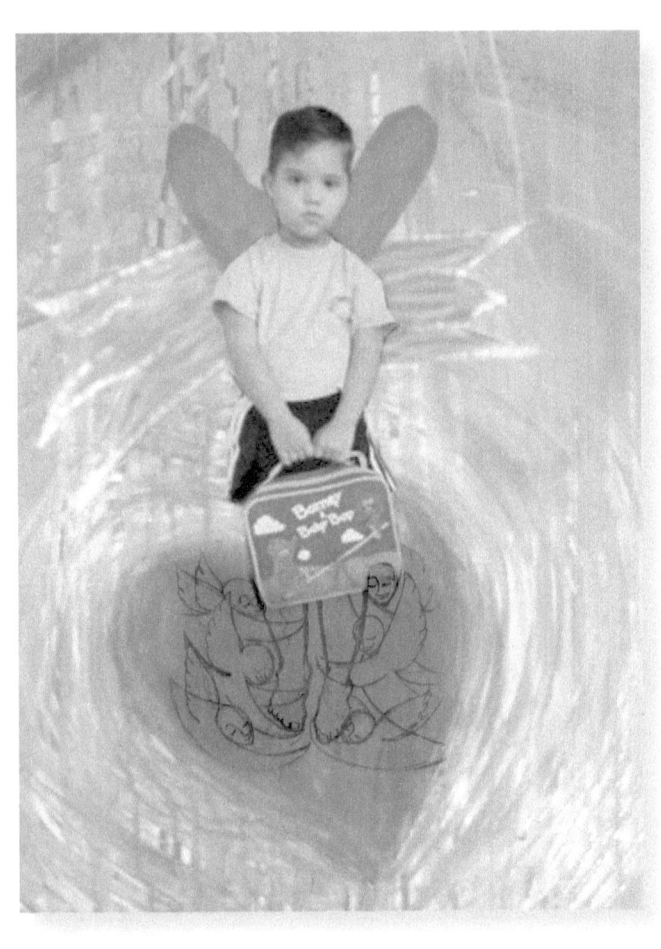

Art by Alexis Artuna

ANGELS

CHAPTER FIVE

Hebrews 1:14

During his process my son discovered angels of light and darkness. Here is how he describes them.

1. Gaby: "God angel is making me a baby"

Hebrews 13:2:
Be not forgetful to entertain strangers: for thereby some have entertained angels unaware.

Mom: Gaby connects with his innocence, his inner child where he feels safe and he describes it as an angel. Maybe he refers to others in helping him to get there.

2. Gaby: "Believe in angels"

Luke 15:10

"Likewise, I say to you, there is joy in the presence of the angels of God over one sinner who repents."

Mom: Gaby seems to feel the presence of angels and the joy this brings.

3. Gaby: "When you sleep, you find your angel"

Genesis 28:12
And he dreamed that there was a ladder set up on the earth, the top of it reaching to heaven; and the angels of God were ascending and descending on it

Mom: Apparently, Gaby has dreams and visions with angels like Jacob did.

4. Gaby: "Angels are around, good angels, not vampire"

Daniel 2:22

Matthew 4:11 Then the devil left him, and angels came and attended him.

Mom: Gaby felt surrounded by good angels.

5. Gaby: "Have you seen angels Gaby?

That's light, sun light, white angels. That's God's angels"

Luke 2:9 An angel of the Lord appeared to them, and the glory of the Lord shine around them, and they were terrified.

Mom: Gaby seems to have seen angels.

6. Gaby: "Angels are protecting"

Hebrews 1:14

Therefore, angels are only servants--spirits sent to care for people who will inherit salvation.

Mom: Gaby felt angels' protection.

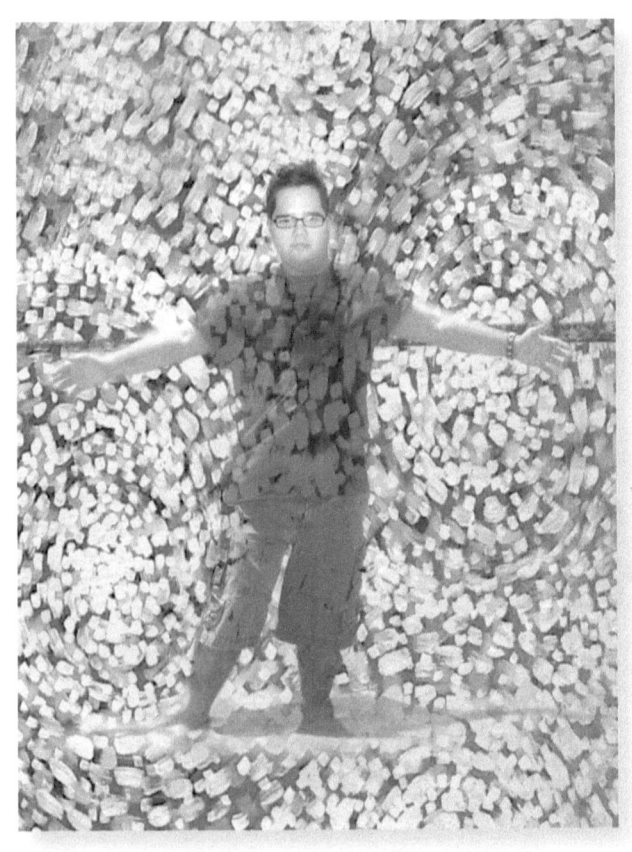

Art by Wilson Romero

<u>FREEDOM</u>

CHAPTER SIX

John 8:36
Gaby's ultimate expression
of freedom from his chains
of sadness, depression, and
confusion.

1. Gaby: "I am free"

John 8:32

Then you will know the truth, and the truth will set you free.

Mom: Gaby encounters freedom when accepting Jesus into his life.

2. Gaby: "My key is Jesus, kingdom of God, freedom"

Corinthians 3:17
Now the Lord is the Spirit, and where the Spirit of the Lord is, there is freedom.

Mom: By accepting Jesus in his heart, Gaby feels he is carrying a key that opens the doorway to God's kingdom.

3. Gaby: "Free bird, white bird"

Galatians 5:1

It is for freedom that Christ has set us free. Stand firm, then, and do not let yourselves be burdened again by a yoke of slavery.

Mom: Gaby feels freed from captivity in his soul like a bird leaving his cage.

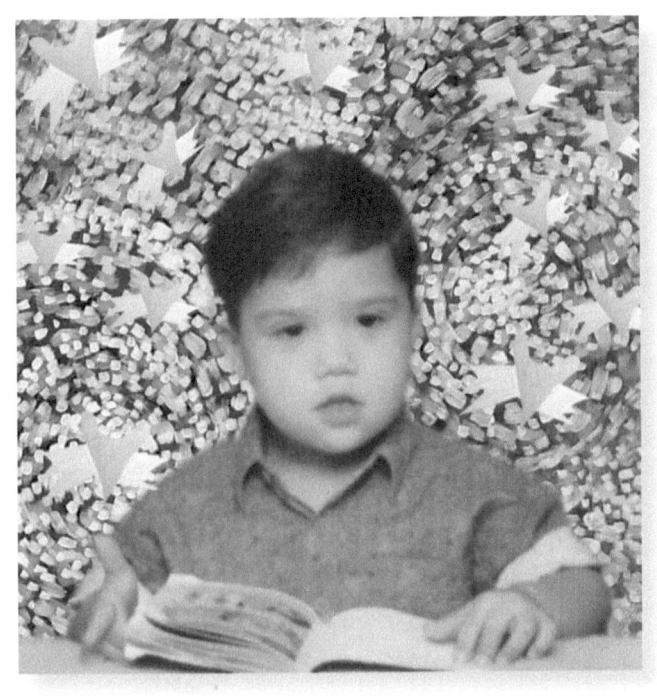

Art by Wilson Romero

RANDOM WISDOM FROM
A PURE HEART

CHAPTER SEVEN

2 Timothy 2:22

Flee the evil desires of youth, and pursue righteousness, faith, love and peace, along with those who call on the Lord out of a pure heart.

Gaby says:

1. "Follow your dream"

2. "I am here for you"

3. "Be free"

4. "Happiness is out there"

5. "Happy is light and the bible"

6. "Friendship is forever never let it go"

7. "I am awake, open the windows in heaven"

8. "I feel great, super, very good"

9. "Everybody loves me, in my heart"

10. "Sadness and crying, you have to pray them"

11. "Everybody says: happy brain and happy heart"

12. "Gaby happy"

13. "I changed for good"

14. "Evil and bad is underground"

15. "Shadow is gone"

16. "I feel open"

17. "Everything is possible"

18. "Family comes first"

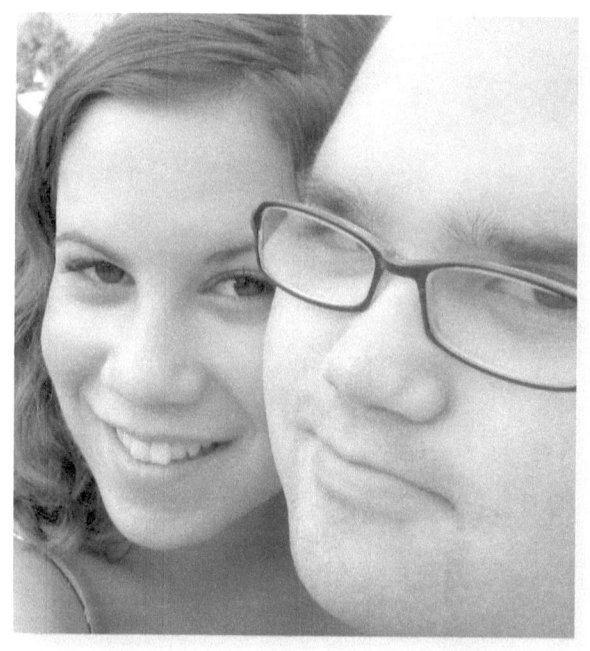

FAMILY COMES FIRST